Rahma Derbel
Jihen Yaich
Salma Ketata

Music therapy and perioperative anxiety

Rahma Derbel
Jihen Yaich
Salma Ketata

Music therapy and perioperative anxiety

ScienciaScripts

Imprint

Any brand names and product names mentioned in this book are subject to trademark, brand or patent protection and are trademarks or registered trademarks of their respective holders. The use of brand names, product names, common names, trade names, product descriptions etc. even without a particular marking in this work is in no way to be construed to mean that such names may be regarded as unrestricted in respect of trademark and brand protection legislation and could thus be used by anyone.

Cover image: www.ingimage.com

This book is a translation from the original published under ISBN 978-620-6-69573-8.

Publisher:
Sciencia Scripts
is a trademark of
Dodo Books Indian Ocean Ltd. and OmniScriptum S.R.L publishing group

120 High Road, East Finchley, London, N2 9ED, United Kingdom
Str. Armeneasca 28/1, office 1, Chisinau MD-2012, Republic of Moldova, Europe
Printed at: see last page
ISBN: 978-620-6-57797-3

CONTENTS

INTRODUCTION

Perioperative anxiety is an unpleasant and common reaction experienced by patients who are scheduled for surgery (1). It is the state of physical and psychological discomfort that patients may feel before and after surgery (2,3). Depending on the study, it affects between 60% and 80% of adults in the operating theatre (4). When the intensity of this anxiety becomes significant, it can meet the criteria for a full-blown panic attack and, in extreme cases, lead to post-traumatic stress disorder.This anxiety is even more apparent during surgery performed under anaesthetic, given that the patient remains conscious during the operation, and especially in the orthopaedic surgery unit, where noise levels are alarmingly high and regularly exceed the limits set by institutional or federal regulations, due to the hammers, drills and oscillating saws frequently used (5). Surgery and anaesthesia are thus generally unpleasant experiences for patients, and are a source of stress and anxiety that can hinder the desired therapeutic objective (6). Indeed, high levels of pre-operative anxiety have been shown to increase the risk of post-operative complications, as well as the occurrence of post-operative emotional and behavioural disorders (2).

To reduce this, sedative or anxiolytic drugs are often administered as premedication before surgery. However, these drugs can be responsible for certain adverse effects that affect patients. For example, higher sedation requirements during hip fracture repair are associated with higher rates of delirium in the elderly population (7).

Furthermore, several recent studies have called into question the benefit of premedication, which does not appear to be superior to placebo (8,9).

For this reason, premedication is increasingly being abandoned and non-pharmacological methods such as music therapy are being developed to improve patients' peri-operative comfort (10).

Traditionally, music has played an important role in human culture and has had a powerful influence on human behaviour. The areas in which music can be used have multiplied with human evolution, including its therapeutic use (11,12). Indeed, both medicine and music can be used to improve the human condition, and their union gives rise to what is known as music therapy. The advent of psychoanalysis in the 20th century gave music its full therapeutic value as a non-pharmacological, inexpensive and risk-free technique. This approach uses the relaxing properties of music to restore, maintain or improve an individual's social, mental and physical capacities (13).

At present, the scientific basis of the effects of music therapy has been the subject of several neurophysiological studies, the results of which have established evidence in particular of the effect of music on hormonal secretions and pain reflexes. However, this harmless tool is not yet well exploited in everyday anaesthetic practice, reflecting the lack of recommendations. This paradoxical situation justifies the need for further studies encouraging the clinical use of music therapy in this field. Hence our interest in evaluating the effect of music therapy on the management of perioperative anxiety in patients proposed for orthopaedic surgery of the lower limb under spinal anaesthesia.

PATIENTS AND METHODS

1. TYPE OF STUDY :

This was a prospective, single-centre, randomised, single-blind clinical trial, carried out in the orthopaedic operating theatre, evaluating the contribution of music therapy during scheduled orthopaedic surgery of the lower limb under spinal anaesthesia (RA). This work was carried out by the team of the anaesthesia and intensive care unit in collaboration with the team of the orthopaedic unit of the CHU Habib BOURGUIBA Sfax and after obtaining informed and signed consent from the patients.

2. STUDY POPULATION :

All patients proposed for scheduled orthopaedic surgery of the lower limb under AR and meeting the following inclusion and exclusion criteria were included in our study:

2.1. Inclusion criteria :

Patients were included in this study:
➤ Age > 18

➤ Classified as ASA I or II by the American Society of Anesthesiology (ASA) (Appendix 1)
➤ Proposed for scheduled orthopaedic surgery of the lower limb under AR
➤ Who agreed to take part in the study.

2.2. Non-inclusion criteria :

➤ Patient refusal to be included in the study

➤ Patients with a known cognitive or psychiatric disorder or who are being monitored by a neurologist or psychiatrist, or who are taking antidepressants or anxiolytics
➤ Patients with age-related hearing loss or hearing loss secondary to illness.

➤ Pregnancy

➤ Misunderstanding the visual analogue scale (VAS) for anxiety and pain

➢ Contraindications to AR:

• Haemostasis disorders

• State of shock

• Uncompensated hypovolaemia

• Unstable arterial hypertension

• Decompensated heart failure

• Tight aortic or mitral stenosis

• Intracranial hypertension

• Infection in the vicinity of the puncture site

• Progressive neurological disease

➢ Allergy to local anaesthetics

➢ The technical difficulties involved in producing AR.

2.3. Exclusion criteria :

➢ Failure of RA requiring conversion to general anaesthesia (GA)

➢ Occurrence of an anaesthetic or surgical complication.

3. DESCRIPTION OF THE STUDY PROTOCOL :

3.1. Anaesthetic consultation :

All patients had an anaesthetic consultation prior to the operation. During this consultation, a standard anaesthetic assessment was carried out.The clinical examination and additional investigations were used to assess the functional reserve of the various organs. Additional tests were requested depending on the patient's condition and the type of surgery. Patients had a chest X-ray and electrocardiogram if necessary.

Theexplorations cardiovascular (including echocardiography thoracic echocardiography) were requested according to the patient's condition. A reserve of packed red blood cells was requested if indicated by the patient's condition and the risk of bleeding during surgery.

3.2. Pre-anaesthetic visit :

During the pre-anaesthetic visit carried out the day before the procedure, the resident checked that the pre-operative instructions given during the anaesthetic consultation had been followed, and then carried out a neurological examination to check for any motor deficit, sensory disability, neurodegenerative disease, hearing impairment, cognitive impairment or any anxiolytic or antidepressant medication being taken, using a simplified questionnaire. It defined the patients eligible for the study by checking the inclusion and non-inclusion criteria. No premedication was administered either the day before or the morning of the procedure.

3.3. Information and consent :

The patient was clearly informed of the anaesthetic protocol and the use of the VAS. The EVA anxiety scale consists of a 10 cm long ruler, the ends of which represent the absence of anxiety on one side (0) and the maximum unimaginable anxiety on the other (10). The patient moves a cursor between the two ends to express the intensity of the anxiety felt. A notation on the back of the ruler is used to assess the anxiety score (Appendix 2). The VAS pain scale consists of a 10 cm long ruler, the ends of which represent the absence of pain on one side (0) and the maximum unimaginable pain on the other (10). The patient moves a cursor between the two ends to indicate the intensity of their pain. A scale on the back of the ruler is used to assess the pain score (Appendix 3). At the end of the pre-anaesthetic visit, an informed consent form was signed by the patients who agreed to take part in the study (Appendix 4).

3.4. Randomisation of groups :

Randomisation was carried out on entry to the operating theatre by an anaesthetist other than the one who would be responsible for data collection and intra- and postoperative follow-up, after verification of the inclusion and non-inclusion criteria. Computerised randomisation software was used to divide patients into two study groups:

- **Study group (M):** patients in this group listened to the music of their choice via headphones during the procedure.
- **Control group (T):** the patients in this group wore headphones without music and were therefore naturally exposed to the sounds of the operating theatre without any isolation.

3.5. Conduct of the study :

• Preoperative :

Socio-demographic parameters and history were recorded. Conditioning and monitoring :
Once the room checklist had been checked, the patient was placed on the operating table.

All patients were monitored by :

- 3-lead electrocardioscope

- Non-invasive blood pressure measurement

- Pulse oximetry.

An 18-gauge peripheral venous line was inserted and filling with 500 cc of 9% saline was started.

Antibiotic prophylaxis :

Antibiotic prophylaxis was taken if indicated. Patients' anxiety was assessed on entry to the operating theatre before the RA procedure, using the VAS Anxiety Scale. The haemodynamic parameters (heart rate (HR), systolic blood pressure (SBP), diastolic blood pressure (DBP) and respiratory rate (RR)) at the start of the procedure were recorded.

● Intraoperative :

Anaesthetic protocol :

The anaesthetic technique used for all patients was AR. The equipment used for AR included:

- A sterile field

- Sterile compresses

- 25 gauge spinal needle with pencil point

- A local anaesthetic: hyperbaric Bupivacaine and a morphine: Fentanyl
- A syringe.

RA was performed in the same way for all patients: The patient was placed in a sitting or lateral position (depending on the patient's tolerance). After rigorous disinfection of the dorsolumbar region, the puncture was made in the L3-L4 or L4-L5 interspinous space. The subarachnoid space was identified by the perceived loss of resistance that preceded the reflux of cerebrospinal fluid. The anaesthetic was injected slowly intrathecally at a rate of 0.1 ml/s.The patient was then returned to a semi-seated position: 30 degree proclivity. Oxygenation was provided using a 4 litre/min flow rate oxygenator.Sensory block was assessed by the thermal method using a compress soaked in ether every two minutes (min) until a metameric level was reached, which was necessary to authorise surgery. If after 20 minutes the level was insufficient, a GA conversion was performed and the patient was excluded from the study.During the installation phase, the engine block was assessed every 5 minutes using the BROMAGE scale (appendix 5), up to a maximum score.

Fitting the helmet :

Patients in the study group (M) chose between 2 types of instrumental music: oriental or classical. These patients then wore headphones attached to an MP3 player with the chosen music.The music began immediately after the patient was settled in following the performance of AR and was maintained until the end of the surgery.The sound volume has been set at 65 decibels, using a telephone application, to avoid any risk of hearing damage from prolonged listening. The tempo of the music was between 60 and 80 beats per minute. Patients in the control group (T) wore headphones without music and were therefore exposed to the noise of the operating theatre. Haemodynamic parameters (HR, SBP, DBP and RF) were recorded every 10 min.Data relating to the surgery (type of surgery, duration of surgery) were recorded. Data relating to anaesthesia (time to sensory and motor block, duration of anaesthesia) were recorded. The doses of ephedrine administered were recorded. No premedication was administered to patients in either group. At the end of the procedure, the MP3 player was switched off and the headphones were removed.

❶ Post-operative :

After the procedure was completed, the patient was transferred to the post-interventional monitoring room (SSPI) for 2 hours to monitor pain, haemodynamic status and side effects. Anxiety levels were re-assessed after the procedure as soon as the patient was admitted to the ICU, using the VAS anxiety scale. Pain levels were also assessed after 2 hours (H2) and then after 6 hours (H6) from the end of the procedure using the pain VAS.

The time taken to administer the first dose of analgesia was also noted. Satisfaction was assessed at the end of the procedure using a Likert scale:

- 1 :very satisfied

- 2 :satisfied

- 3 :undetermined

- 4: not satisfied

Patients were asked if they wanted to repeat the procedure using the same protocol and answered with:

- Yes

- No

4. PARAMETERS COLLECTED :

The data collection form included (appendix 6):

4.1. Pre-operatively on entry to the operating theatre:

- The patient's socio-demographic characteristics: age, sex, level of education, marital status, co-morbidities, ASA class, weight, height, body mass index (BMI), etc.
- Assessing anxiety using the EVA anxiety scale

- Haemodynamic parameters (HR, SAP, DBP and RF)

- Music group (M) or control group (T)

- The music chosen by the patients in the M.

4.2. Intraoperative :

- Haemodynamic parameters (HR, PAS, PAD, FR) every 10 minutes.

- Type of surgery (total knee replacement (TKR), meniscus surgery, ligamentoplasty, removal of material, other: lipoma or synovial cyst)
- Duration of surgery

- The time taken to install the sensory block

- The time taken to install the engine block

- The duration of the anaesthetic.

4.3. Post-operative :

- EVA anxiety

- Pain VAS at H2 and H6 post-op

- Time to first analgesic intake

- Patient satisfaction

- Patients' choice to repeat the procedure using the same protocol.

5. JUDGING CRITERIA :

5.1. Primary endpoint:

The primary endpoint was to evaluate the effectiveness of music therapy in managing perioperative anxiety.

5.2. Secondary endpoints :

The secondary endpoints were to evaluate :

- Post-operative pain

- Intraoperative haemodynamic stability

- Patient satisfaction.

6. STATISTICAL STUDY :

6.1. Sample calculation :

The number of patients required was determined from the results of a pre-survey of 20 patients. Assuming a two-tailed test power of 90% and an alpha risk of 5%, the number of patients required was 18 per group. We then designated 54 patients per group to ensure a sufficient number after possible exclusions.

6.2. Statistical analysis :

The data were analysed using SPSS software version 26.0. We checked the normality of the distributions using the Shapiro- test. Wilk.For the descriptive study, the qualitative variables were expressed as numbers and percentages and the quantitative variables as mean +/- standard deviation. in the case of a normal distribution and the median with its extremes in the opposite case.For the comparative study, qualitative variables were tested using the chi-square test (or Fisher's exact test if the number < 5). Quantitative variables were tested using the Student's t-test in the case of a normal distribution and the Mann Whitney U-test in the case of an abnormal distribution. The significance threshold was set at 0.05.

RESULTS

The study was conducted over a 1-year period from 1er January 2022 to 31 May 2023. One hundred and eight patients were included in our work and were divided into two equivalent groups. Two patients were excluded from the

T. One patient was excluded because the duration of surgery exceeded the duration of anaesthesia requiring GA conversion, and another patient was excluded because of AR failure. Two patients in group M were excluded due to failure of RA. The number of subjects selected was 104, with 52 subjects in each group.

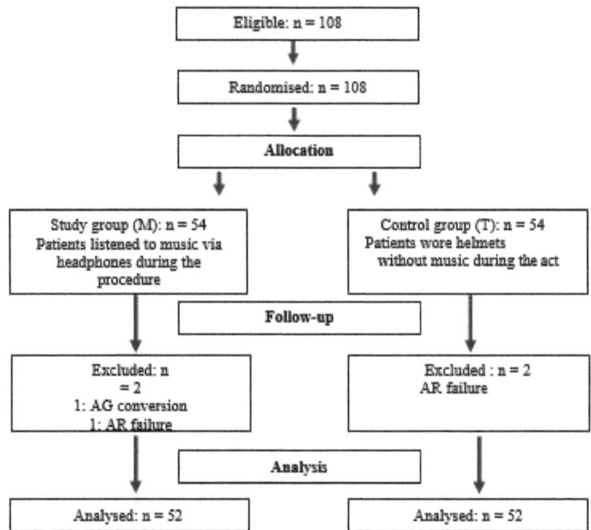

T: control, M: music, RA: rachi anaesthesia, AG: general anaesthesia
Figure 1: Flow chart

1. DEMOGRAPHIC PARAMETERS :

The median age of the study population was 65 [22-88].The sample comprised 49 women and 55 men, with a sex ratio (M/F) of 1.12. The mean BMI was 27.963 ± 4.506 kg/cm².Demographic parameters were statistically comparable between the two groups **(Table I)**.

Table I: Comparison of demographic parameters between the two groups.

	Group T (n = 52)	Group M (n = 52)	p
Age (years) (median+ interval)	66,5 [22-82]	63 [22-83]	0,410§
Weight (kg) (mean ± SD)	78,50 ± 12,417	76,02 ± 9,807	0,261*
Height (cm) (mean ± SD)	1,67 ± 0,747	1,68 ± 0,760	0,938*
BMI (kg/cm²) (median + range)	28,72 [20,20-41,91]	26,51 [20,06-37,11]	0,088§
Gender (M/F)	28/24	27/25	0,844 †

***: student's t test, †: chi-square test, §: Mann Whitney test, n: number of patients, SD: standard deviation, T: control, M: music, BMI: body mass index, Kg: kilogram, cm: centimetre, M: man, F: woman.**

We have not noted any difference significant difference in the marital status between the 2 groups **(table II)**.

Table II: Comparison of marital status between the two groups.

	Group T (n = 52)	Group M (n = 52)	p
Married	28 (53,8%)	27 (51,9%)	
Divorced	5 (9,6%)	7 (13,5%)	
			0,642†
Single	6 (11,5%)	9 (17,3%)	
Widower	13 (25%)	9 (17,3%)	

†: chi-square test, n: number of patients, T: control, M: music

Educational levels were statistically comparable between the 2 groups **(Table III)**.

Table III: Comparison of educational levels between the two groups.

	Group T (n = 52)	Group M (n = 52)	p
Illiterate	16 (30,8%)	11 (21,2%)	
Primary	16 (30,8%)	15 (28,8%)	
			0,604†
Secondary	14 (26,9%)	17 (32,7%)	
University	6 (11,5%)	9 (17,3%)	

†: chi-square test, n: number of patients, T: control, M: music

2. COMORBIDITES :

The main comorbidities found in both groups are summarised in **Figure 2**.

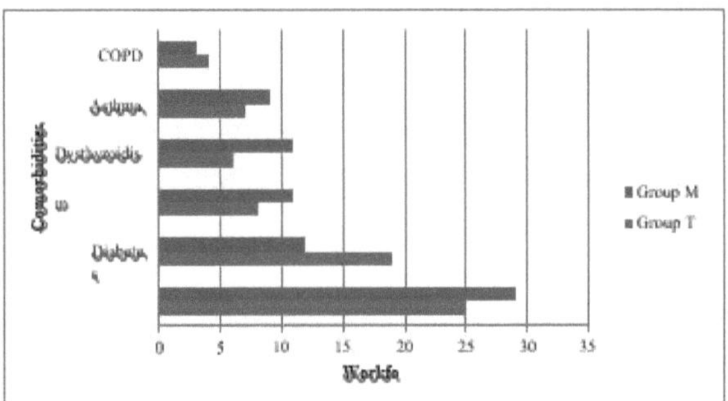

**T: control, M: music, COPD: chronic obstructive pulmonary disease,
Stroke: Cerebrovascular accident, HTA: High blood pressure**
Figure 2: Distribution of patients by comorbidity between the two groups.

According to the ASA classification, 34 patients in group T and 28 patients in group M were classified as ASA II, i.e. 65.38% and 53.84% of cases respectively. There was no statistically significant difference in ASA status between the two groups **(Table VI)**.

Table IV: Comparison of ASA classification between the two groups.

	Group T (n = 52)	Group M (n = 52)	p
ASA I	18 (34,61%)	24 (46,15%)	0,318†
ASA II	34 (65,38%)	28 (53,84%)	

†: chi-square test, n: number of patients, T: control, M: music, ASA: American society of anesthesiologists

3. CHOICE OF MUSIC :

Eighty-two per cent of patients in group M chose oriental instrumental music **(Figure 3).**

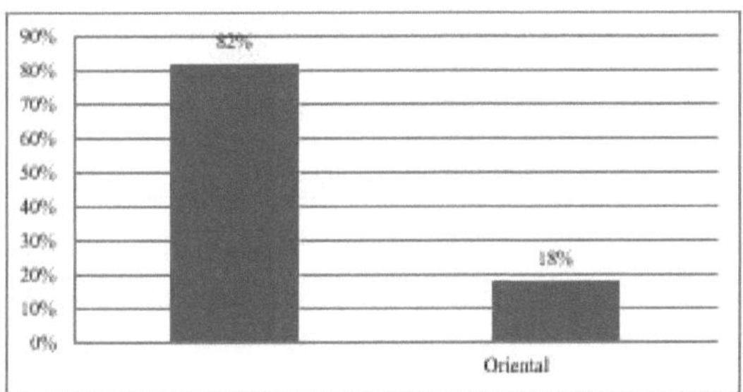

Figure 3: Breakdown of Group M by music chosen

4. PARAMETERS RELATING TO SURGERY :

4.1. Type of surgery :

There was no statistically significant difference in the type of surgery between the 2 groups (p = 0.841) **(Figure 4).**

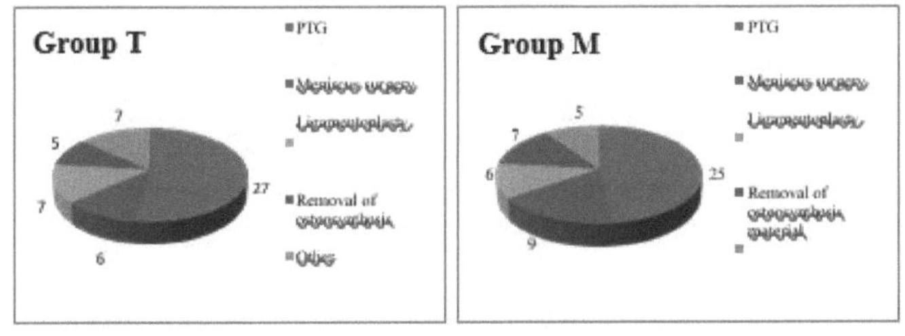

T: control, M: music, PTG: total knee prosthesis
Figure 4: Distribution of patients by type of surgery.

4.2. Duration of surgery :

There was no significant difference between the two groups in the duration of surgery **(Table V).**

Table V: Comparison of the duration of surgery between the two groups.

	Group T	Group M	p
Average duration of surgery (min) (mean ± SD)	97.11 ± 5.10	98.62 ± 4.15	0 ,818*

*: student's t test, SD: standard deviation, T: control, M: music, mn: minute

5. PARAMETERS RELATING TO ANAESTHESIA :

5.1. Installation time for the sensory and motor unit :

Sensory block was obtained on average after more than 5 minutes in both groups. There was no significant difference between the two groups in the time taken to achieve sensory block (p=0.154). The motor block was obtained within the first 10 minutes after RA in both groups. There was no significant difference between the two groups in the time taken to install the motor block (p=0.183).

5.2. Duration of anaesthesia :

There was no significant difference between the two groups in the duration of anaesthesia **(table VI).**

Table VI: Comparison of duration of anaesthesia between the two groups.

	Group T	Group M	p
Average duration of anaesthesia (min) (mean ± SD)	159.58 ± 8.88	160.60 ± 9.17	0.53*

*: student's t test, SD: standard deviation, T: control, M: music, mn: minute

6. VISUAL ANALOG SCALE OF ANXIETY :

Preoperatively, there was no significant difference in VAS anxiety scores between the two groups. The mean preoperative VAS anxiety score was 5.33 ±

2.130 in group T and 5.23 ± 2.32 in group M (p = 0.655) **(Figure 5)**. Post-operatively, we noted that the mean VASanxiety scores were statistically significantly lower in the M group than in the T group. The mean postoperative VAS anxiety score was 2.94 ± 1.364 in group T, and 1.83 ± 0.760 in group M, (p < 0.001) **(Figure 5)**.

T: control, M: music, VAS: visual analogue scale

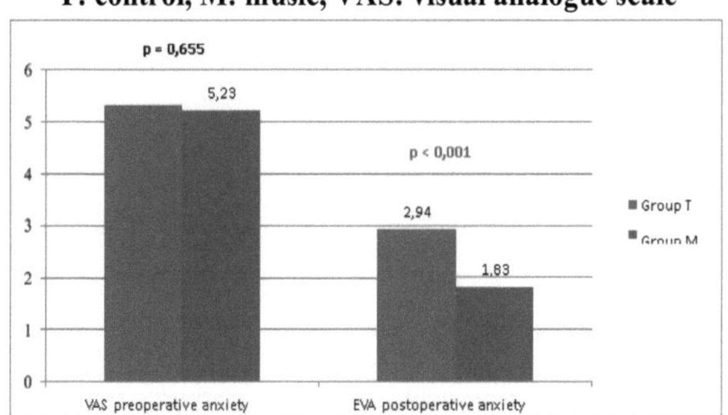

Figure 5: Comparison of the means of the VAS anxiety scores for pre- and post-op between the two groups.

7. PAIN AND INITIAL ANALGESIC INTAKE :

7.1. Visual analogue pain scale :

Comparison of pain VAS values at H2 and H6 post-op between the two groups showed a significant difference in favour of group M over group T (p<0.001) **(Figure 6)**.

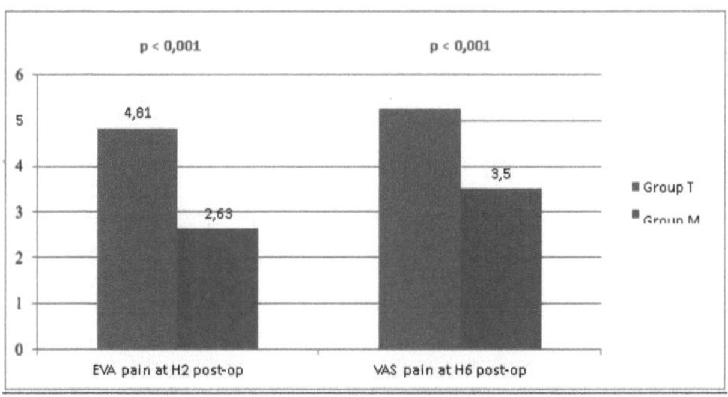

T: control, M: music, VAS: visual analogue scale

Figure 6: Comparison of mean VAS scores for postoperative pain between the two groups.

7.2. Time to first analgesic :

The use of postoperative analgesia was statistically significantly earlier in patients in group T than in group M (p<0.001) (**Table VII**).

Table VII: Comparison of mean time to first analgesic between the two groups.

	Group T	Group M	P
Deadline of analgesic (min) (mean ± SD)	158,22 ± 25,762	242,1 ± 29,154	<0,001*

***: student's t test, SD: standard deviation, T: control, M: music, mn: minute**

8. HEMODYNAMIC PARAMETERS :

8.1. Heart rate :

The mean heart rate measured preoperatively was 91.63 ± 7.25 in group T and 89.26 ± 8.85 in group M.No significant difference between the two groups was observed when HR was measured pre-operatively (p= 0.120). We noted a significant difference between the two groups at all times of intraoperative HR measurement (p<0.05), except at the tenth minute (T10) when we did not note a significant difference in HR between the 2 groups **(Figure 7).**

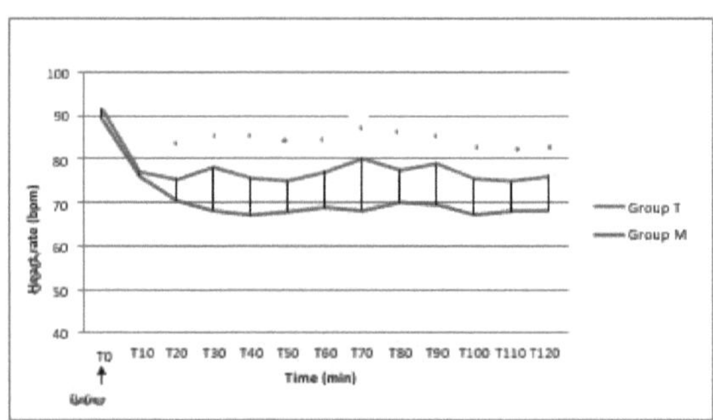

T: control; M: music; bpm: beats per minute; mn: minutes, RA: anaesthesia rachi, *: p < 0.05

Figure 7: Evolution of average heart rates intraoperatively.

8.2. Blood pressure :

The mean values of PAS and PAD observed preoperatively were comparable in the two groups.The mean preoperative SBP was 143.54 ± 2.21 millimetres of mercury (mmHg) in group T and 140.78 ± 2.53 mmHg in group M. The mean preoperative DBP was 78.54 ± 12.85 mmHg in group T and 76.69 ± 12.91 mmHg in group M.Pre-operatively, there was no significant difference between the two groups in the measurement of PAS (p = 0.322) and PAD (p = 0.154) **(Figure 8)**.The mean SAP and DBP values observed intraoperatively were comparable in the two groups.Nous n'avons pas trouvé une différence significative entre les deux groupes à chacun des moments de mesure des pressions artérielles en per opératoire (p>0,05) bien que les valeurs de la PAS et PAD soient inférieures dans le groupe M que dans le groupe T à tous les temps de mesure **(Figure 8)**.

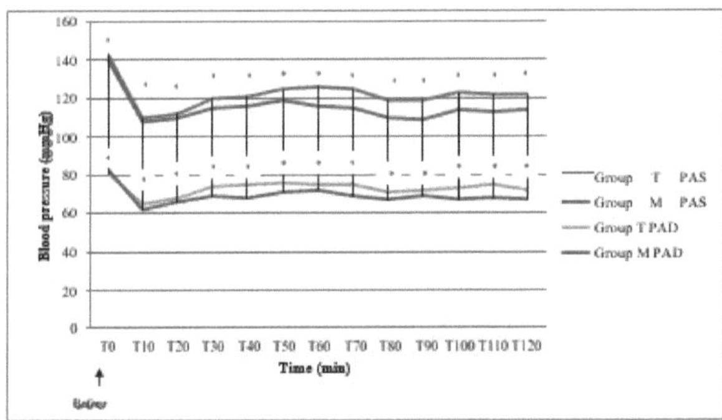

T: control; M: music; mmHg: millimetre of mercury; mn: minutes, RA: anaesthetic patch, SBP: systolic blood pressure, DBP: diastolic blood pressure, *: p > 0.05

Figure 8: Changes in mean systolic and diastolic blood pressure during the operation.

8.3. Respiratory rate :

The mean RF measured preoperatively was 21.12 ± 2.54 cycles per minute (cpm) in group T and 22.64 ± 2.41 cpm in group M.There was no significant difference between the two groups when FRs were measured preoperatively (p = 0.215).The mean respiratory rates observed intraoperatively were comparable in the two groups, and we did not find a significant difference between the two groups at each of the times at which respiratory rates were measured intraoperatively, except at T60 and T80 where we found a significant difference between the 2 groups.In addition, the mean respiratory frequencies measured at all times were lower in group M than in group T **(Figure 9)**.

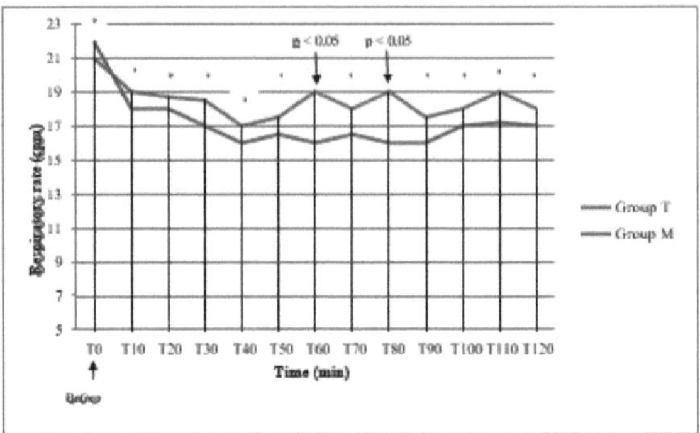

T: control; M: music; cpm: cycles per minute; mn: minutes, RA: anaesthesia rachi, *: p>0.05

Figure 9: Changes in mean respiratory frequency during surgery.

8.4. Ephedrine doses :

Mean ephedrine doses ranged from 0 to 30 milligrams (mg) in both groups. There was no significant difference between the two groups in the dose of ephedrine administered **(Table VIII)**.

Table VIII: Comparison of the mean dose of ephedrine administered in the two study groups

	Group T	Group M	P
Ephedrine dose (mg)	4,5[0-30]	6[0-30]	0,819§

§: Mann Whitney test, [ ]: extremes, T: control, M: music, mg: milligram

9. PATIENT SATISFACTION :

Post-operatively, the satisfaction rate of group M was significantly higher than that of group T **(Table IX)**.

Table IX: Distribution of patients according to their postoperative satisfaction levels

	Group T	Group M	P
Very satisfied	8 (15,38%)	21 (40,1%)	
Satisfied	15 (28,84%)	24 (46,2%)	
Undetermined	18 (34,61%)	7 (13,5%)	< 0,001†
Not satisfied	11 (21,15%)	0 (0%)	

† : chi-squared test

When asked if they wanted to repeat the procedure using the same protocol, 49 patients in group M (94.2%) said yes, compared with 29 patients in group T (55.8%). This difference was highly significant in favour of group M (p < 0.001).Three patients in the group answeredno to the question. They said they would have preferred to listen to the Koran.

DISCUSSION

We conducted a single-blind, prospective, randomised controlled trial including patients proposed for scheduled orthopaedic surgery of the lower limb under AR.One hundred and four patients were included and randomised into two groups of 52 :

- Study group (M): patients in this group listened to the music of their choice via headphones during the procedure.

- Control group (T): the patients in this group wore headphones without music and were therefore naturally exposed to the sounds of the operating theatre without any isolation.

Socio-demographic parameters, ASA score, type of surgery, duration of surgery, time to onset of sensory and motor block and duration of anaesthesia were comparable between the two groups. Preoperative VAS anxiety scores were comparable between the two groups. However, postoperatively, these scores were statistically significantly lower in group M than in group T.Post-operative pain VAS values at H2 and H6 were statistically significantly lower in group M than in group T. The use of postoperative analgesia was statistically significantly earlier in patients in group T than in group M.Intraoperatively, we noted a significant difference between the two groups at all times of intraoperative HR measurement, except at T10 when we did not note a significant difference in HR between the 2 groups. There was no statistically significant difference between the two groups in terms of variations in PAS and PAD intraoperatively, although there was a significant difference in PAS and PAD between the two groups. PAS and PAD values were lower in group M at all measurement times. We did not find a significant difference between the two groups at each of the times at which respiratory rates were measured intraoperatively, except at T60 and T80 where we found a significant difference between the 2 groups. In addition, the mean respiratory rates measured at all time points were lower in group M than in group T. Post-operatively, the satisfaction rate of group M was significantly higher than that of group T

1. PERIOPERATIVE ANXIETY :

Perioperative anxiety refers to a state of physical and psychological discomfort that patients may experience before and after surgery (2). High levels of pre-operative anxiety have been shown to increase the risk of post-operative complications, as well as the occurrence of post-operative emotional and behavioural disorders (3). Certain physiological manifestations appear, such as a change in voice (higher pitched), increased heart rate and respiratory rate, shivering and trembling (2,3). The risk factors for peri-operative anxiety are cancer, smoking, psychiatric disorders (anxiety and depressive disorders in particular), moderate to severe pre-operative pain, major surgery and being female (14). Several other factors are responsible for increasing perioperative anxiety, in particular noise in the operating theatre.Noise in the operating theatre is recognised as a source of psychological stress and anxiety for patients. The World Health Organisation (WHO) recommends that noise levels should not exceed 35 decibels (15).However, noise levels in the operating theatre are alarming and regularly exceed the limits set by institutional or federal regulations (16,17). Orthopaedic surgery units are, by their very nature, always very noisy: plaster saws and surgical motors (80 to 90 dB), cups falling to the floor (>90 dB), handling of surgical containers (80 dB) and scopes alarms (50 to 70 dB) (18). In 2007, a study by Kracht et al in the operating theatres of the Johns Hopkins Hospital found that noise levels in orthopaedics exceeded 100 dB for more than 40% of the operating time (5). In addition, the alarm sound of the respirator, scope and syringe pumps, the checking of equipment by the anaesthetic team, the opening of bags and the opening of drawers in the anaesthetic trolley are a source of stress and anxiety for the patient (5).

2. THE BENEFITS OF MUSIC THERAPY :

2.1. In medicine :

Music therapy (MT) has been widely used in various health sectors. Music is a very old therapeutic method whose effectiveness has been proven mainly in the treatment of physical and mental stress linked to certain neuropsychiatric disorders, in the treatment of cancer, in surgical interventions and in several other health sectors.To evaluate the effects of music-based therapeutic interventions for people with dementia, in 2017, in Spain, M. Gómez Gallego et al conducted a study on 42 patients with mild to moderate Alzheimer's disease. These patients followed a TM protocol for 6 weeks. Each session included several activities: songs with background music, song recognition games, dancing, etc. The activity was designed and carried out by 2 professionals trained in TM.Changes in the results of the mini-mental state examination, the neuropsychiatric inventory, the Hospital Anxiety and Depression scale and Barthel index scores were studied. TM considerably increased the mini-mental state examination score, particularly in the areas of orientation, language and memory. An improvement in certain cognitive, psychological and behavioural changes was also noted in patients with Alzheimer's disease (19).For children with autism, TM has been shown to improve communication skills and also parent-child relationships (20). In 2018 in Montreal Canada, 51 children aged 6 to 12 years with autism were randomised into 2 groups, a control group and a TM group where patients received 8 to 12 weeks of musical intervention. The musical intervention involved the use of improvisational approaches through singing and rhythm to target social communication. The non-musical intervention was based on structurally adapted behavioural management implemented in a non-musical context. This study provides the first evidence that 8 to 12 weeks of individual music intervention can indeed improve social communication and functional brain connectivity (21).A meta-analysis was conducted in 2019 in China to evaluate the effectiveness of TM on quality of life, anxiety, depression and pain in cancer patients. A total of 1,548 patients were included in the study, 765 in the control group and 783 in the study group. TM significantly improved the overall quality of life scores of cancer patients. Anxiety, depression and pain scores were also significantly reduced in the study group (22).The growing use of TM in the delivery room is showing encouraging results in terms of anxiety and pain, particularly in primiparous women.(23). The results revealed significant differences in VAS scores for anxiety and pain in the use of TM in the latent phase and in the active phase of labour. Similarly, one study evaluated differences in anxiety levels measured with a VAS during the postpartum period in primiparous patients, finding significant differences in favour of the TM group, one hour to 24 hours after delivery (24).

2.2. In the operating theatre :

To reduce perioperative anxiety, sedative or anxiolytic drugs are usually administered as premedication before surgery (8). However, these drugs may be responsible for adverse effects that can affect patient discharge, particularly in outpatient surgery. These drugs can depress the respiratory and circulatory systems. In addition, several recent studies have called into question the value of premedication, whose efficacy does not appear to be greater than that of a placebo (8). The systematic administration of premedication is therefore currently tending to diminish, while non-medicinal approaches such as TM or hypnosis are tending to develop to improve patients' pre-operative comfort (1,10). TM, as a non-medicinal intervention, has shown positive effects on perioperative anxiety and has made it possible to achieve haemodynamic stability intraoperatively (25). The value of music therapy has also been demonstrated in GA surgery, where an improvement in pain scores and patient satisfaction has been noted (26,27). The mechanism by which TM reduces the perception of pain and anxiety is by modifying the electrical activity of the brain during the stressful event (28). Musical intervention also distracts patients from their environment. It can act as an isolator from the noises in the operating theatre that cause anxiety and stress, such as the beeping of instruments, conversations in the operating theatre and the surgeon's orders. (29). The combination of relaxation, distraction and isolation from surrounding noise achieved with TM can improve perceived pain and help patients cope with anxiety (30).

3. CHOICE OF MUSIC :

The pieces of music with the greatest potential for relaxation embody several characteristics. A tempo of 60 to 80 beats per minute, the same as the adult human heart rate, is considered soothing (31). Music suitable for reducing anxiety has a slow, stable rhythm, low-frequency tones, orchestral effects and soothing, relaxing melodies (31). A study by the Bettermann team (32) showed that there is a similarity between the heartbeat and the composition of African music. It showed that the rhythm of the heartbeat, particularly during nocturnal sleep, can be interpreted as a musical rhythm. The heartbeat follows a cycle that can be likened to a piece of music. This property may explain the effect of music on heart rate regulation.

4. DISCUSSION OF OUR RESULTS :

4.1. Anxiety :

In our study, anxiety was assessed by the VAS, which correlates with STAI 7 (33).The VAS anxiety scores were comparable between the two groups preoperatively. Post-operatively, these scores were significantly lower in group M than in group T.Similar results have been published in the literature despite the use of different tools to assess the degree of stress felt by the patient. In Brazil in 2021, Azi et al conducted a single-centre, prospective, randomised controlled trial on patients proposed for orthopaedic surgery of the lower limb under AR. This study showed a significant reduction in anxiety scores assessed by the STAI post-operatively in patients who listened to instrumental music via headphones during surgery (34). Kaur et al conducted a study in 2022 on 70 patients proposed for elective orthopaedic surgery of the lower limb under AR.

A statistically significant difference in VAS scores for intraoperative and postoperative anxiety in favour of the TM group was noted (35).In March 2020, in the USA, Kukreja et al conducted a randomised controlled trial to study the value of TM during PTG surgery under AR. This study showed a reduction in the need for sedation in the TM group. Also, patients in the TM group had lower postoperative STAI anxiety scores than those in the control group (36).In 2014 in China, Wang et al conducted a randomised trial on elderly patients proposed for elective gynaecological or orthopaedic surgery, to assess the effect of listening to music for 30 minutes before surgery on patients' anxiety, assessed by the Zung Self-Rating Anxiety Scale. The anxiety score in these patients decreased significantly after surgery, unlike the control group where the anxiety score remained unchanged (37). In 2018, a meta-analysis of 72 studies involving 7,000 patients and looking at different TM practices showed a reduction in anxiety and postoperative pain in patients receiving musical interventions before, during or after surgery. The effect was most marked when TM was used postoperatively and the patient was able to choose what he or she wanted to listen to from a predefined list of pieces. The effect, which was also noted under GA, was nevertheless slightly greater when patients were conscious during the operation (38).In Turkey, in 2020, Cimen et al carried out a randomised study on 41 patients proposed for arteriovenous fistula surgery under local anaesthetic to study the effect of TM on anxiety levels and perceived pain. Post-operative anxiety levels measured by the STAI were significantly lower in the TM group, where patients listened to music throughout the procedure (39).In China, in 2013, a randomised study was carried out by Zhang et al on male patients proposed for cystoscopy under local anaesthesia, to assess the impact of listening to favourite music during the procedure on patients' pain and anxiety relief. This study showed a statistically significantly lower reduction in the STAI score in the TM group after the procedure than in the control group (P < 0.001) (40).In Taiwan in 2017, Wu et al conducted an experimental study on patients proposed for awake craniotomy to investigate the effect of listening to favourite music in the waiting room and throughout surgery on perioperative anxiety. Patients in the control group showed no difference in anxiety scores measured by the STAI before and after surgery. Patients in the music group had significantly lower scores after 30 minutes of MT, in contrast to the control group where the pre- and postoperative anxiety scores showed no difference (25). In 2005, a study assessed the effect of music therapy on haemodynamic and respiratory parameters, arousal-vigilance and pain in intensive care patients. After randomisation, patients received either a 20-minute MT session of their choice or a 20-minute rest session. This study showed that TM reduced anxiety and pain and led to relaxation in a comparable way in non-intubated and intubated resuscitation patients undergoing ventilatory weaning (41).In 2020, a systematic review and meta-analysis was carried out by Santivañez-Acosta et al, to assess the effectiveness of TM in managing anxiety in pregnant women during labour. VAS anxiety scores decreased in both the latent and active phases of labour (23).

4.2. Pain :

Preoperative anxiety is a predictor of greater postoperative pain. A meta-analysis of the literature published in the American Society of Anesthesiologists in 2009 identified 15 studies showing a significant correlation between pre-operative anxiety and post-operative pain (42).In our study, pain was assessed using the pain VAS. Comparison of VAS pain values at H2 and H6 post-op between the two groups showed a significant difference in favour of the M group compared with the T group.Similar results have been published in the literature. Studies evaluating music in healthcare settings do not necessarily distinguish TM performed by a music therapist from simply listening to background music or music chosen by the patient according to his or her taste. There is a dose effect of TM in reducing pain (24).In China in 2013, a randomised study carried out by Zhang et al on male patients proposed for cystoscopy under local anaesthetic showed that the VAS pain scores after the procedure were significantly lower in the TM group than in the control group (40).In 2013, in Rome, Angioli et al conducted a study on 356 women proposed for live hysteroscopy to investigate the effect of listening to favourite music during the procedure on anxiety and pain perception. A significant reduction in VAS pain scores during and after the procedure was noted in the TM group (43).

In 2019 in Turkey, a randomised study was carried out by Gökçek and kaydu on 120 patients proposed for elective septorhinoplasty under GA. All patients underwent GA with IOT. Patients in the TM group wore headphones and listened to their favourite music during surgery and patients in the control group received usual care without music. In the TM group, VAS pain scores were significantly lower than in the control group (p<0.001), requiring less analgesic medication (17).In March 2018, Gallagher et al conducted a randomised controlled trial on 163 patients proposed for elective orthopaedic surgery of the lower limb. Patients were randomised into a TM group where patients participated in TM sessions within 24 hours of admission, as well as every day of their stay for 30 minutes, and a control group where patients received standard medical care. The TM sessions included listening to favourite music, singing, improvisation on instruments and music-assisted relaxation techniques. There was a significant reduction in VAS pain scores in the MT group compared with the control group. A decrease of at least 2 points in the VAS pain score was noted in 36% of the M group and 10% of the T group (p < 0.001). Seventy-three per cent of M patients compared with 41% of T patients reported an improvement in pain (p<0.001) (44).

4.3. Haemodynamic profile :

In our study, our results showed that MT provided better intraoperative HR stability. We noted a significant difference between the two groups at all times of intraoperative HR measurement, except at the tenth minute (T10) when we did not note a significant difference in HR between the 2 groups. However, we did not show a statistically significant difference in PAS, PAD and RF between the 2 groups.This was consistent with studies in the literature, and inconsistent with other studies.Kaur et al conducted a study in 2022 on 70 patients proposed for elective orthopaedic surgery of the lower limb under AR. HR was comparable in the music (M) and control (C) groups at baseline and after 5 minutes of assessment. Thereafter, HR was lower in the M group throughout the intraoperative period. The difference was statistically significant after 10 minutes and statistically significant (p<0.001) for the remainder of the period. There was no significant difference in mean arterial pressure values intraoperatively between the 2 groups. After 5 minutes from the start of surgery, there was a statistically significant reduction in RF in group M compared with group C (35). In Turkey, in 2020, Cimen et al carried out a randomised study on 41 patients proposed for arteriovenous fistula surgery under local anaesthetic, which showed that the preoperative haemodynamic parameters (PAS, PAD, HR, oxygen saturation and RF) showed no significant difference between the control group and the MT group. However, postoperatively, all these parameters showed significant differences between the two groups, in favour of the MT group where all these values were lower than in the control group (39). In 2016 in Sousse, Tunisia, Kahloul et al conducted a prospective, randomised, double-blind study in the visceral surgery operating theatre on patients proposed for scheduled surgery under GA. Comparison of the haemodynamic profile between the two groups found better haemodynamic stability only for PAS in the MT group where patients listened to music during the actosurgery, but not for PAD and mean arterial pressure, where the two groups were comparable (26). To investigate the effects of TM on haemodynamic parameters in patients proposed for awake craniotomy, an experimental study was conducted by Wu et al in

Taiwan in 2017. This study showed that in patients in the TM group who listened to preferred music preoperatively and intraoperatively, a significant decrease in HR, SBP and DBP preoperatively and intraoperatively during surgery was noted. RF showed no significant difference (25).In 2005 in France, a study carried out by Jaber et al on 30 non-sedated, non-intubated or intubated resuscitation patients undergoing respiratory weaning, showed that a 20-minute music therapy session resulted in a significant reduction in HR, SBP and RF (41).Steelma conducted a study on the effect of instrumental music on blood pressure in patients proposed for hand or wrist surgery under local or locoregional anaesthesia. This study showed that in patients who listened to music during the procedure, there was a statistically significant reduction in PAS and PAD postoperatively (45).In 2013, a study carried out in Rome by Angiolini et al on 356 women proposed for live hysteroscopy showed that during the procedure, PAS and HR were significantly lower in the MT group, where patients listened to music during the procedure, compared with the control group (43).These haemodynamic effects of music can be explained by the fact that music decreases the levels of several hormones and biochemical markers of stress such as cortisol, epinephrine and noradrenaline, due to the neuronal interconnections of the auditory pathway with the hypothalamus and hippocampus (46). The auditory interconnections in the hypothalamus, hippocampus and reticular activating system attenuate the release of excitatory neurotransmitters that are responsible for the sedative and relaxing effects of music (47). This diverts attention away from negative stimuli and focuses the patient's awareness on the music (48). Music contains rhythms and melodies that help individuals to achieve a state of peace, relieve the patient's discomfort and maintain and promote health of the body and mind (5). Music affects the limbic system, which regulates deep emotions and many autonomic parameters. It has been postulated that music causes the body to release its own endorphins, thereby reducing pain and the need for analgesics (47). Music thus appears to have a positive effect on regulating heart rate and on the stress that leads to hypertensive peaks.

4.4. SATISFACTION :

In our study, the patient satisfaction rate was statistically significantly higher in group M. When asked if they wanted to repeat the procedure using the same protocol, 49 patients in group M (94.2%) said yes, compared with 29 patients in group T (55.8%). This difference was highly significant in favour of group M (p

< 0.001). Similar results have been published in the literature (28,36,49). In March 2020, in the USA, Kukreja et al conducted a randomised controlled trial on the effects of TM during PTG surgery under RA. Satisfaction scores were higher in the TM group, where patients listened to music intraoperatively. These patients also indicated that they would ask to listen to music intraoperatively in the future and that they would recommend it to family and friends. Sixty-nine per cent of the control group wanted music to be played (36).In 2018 in Turkey, a randomised study by Bashiri et al on adult patients proposed for colonoscopy showed that patients who listened to music during the procedure were less anxious, were satisfied with their procedure and stated that they would prefer to listen to music during their next endoscopy (28).In 2019 in Turkey, a randomised study was carried out by Gökçek and kaydu on 120 patients proposed for elective septorhinoplasty under GA. All patients underwent GA with IOT. Patient satisfaction was significantly higher in the music group, where patients listened to music during the procedure, than in the control group (73.3% versus 36.6%).%) (49).

5. STRENGTHS AND LIMITATIONS OF THE STUDY :

5.1. Highlights of the study :

This was a prospective randomised controlled trial involving a diverse orthopaedic population.Our results are encouraging and support the use of MT in patients proposed for scheduled lower limb surgery under AR. TM is a simple, effective technique that offers a number of advantages, is inexpensive, feasible in our hospitals and risk-free, making it easy to implement in our operating theatres.

5.2. Limitations of the study :

It was impossible to carry out the study with the same operator, as the clinical trial took place in a university hospital centre where resident and senior surgeons operate together. Anxiety was not assessed using the STAI 7. This scale is in the form of a 40-question questionnaire, comprising two separate parts of twenty questions each for state anxiety and trait anxiety. The patient is asked to answer 20 questions in each part, each response being on a 4-point Likert scale. It was difficult to use this test for our patients, the majority of whom are illiterate and therefore unable to fill in the Arabic version of the questionnaire. Assessing postoperative pain is a difficult task, for reasons that have to do with the highly personal nature of the pain sensation and its interaction with affective and cognitive elements, which are often in the foreground. The inter-individual variability of pain perception is also a major limitation of our study. On the other hand, the social environment and religious beliefs that do not allow music can hamper the effectiveness of TM.

CONCLUSION

Perioperative anxiety is a frequent phenomenon among patients. It is even more apparent in patients undergoing surgery in an operating theatre, and especially in the orthopaedic unit, where noise levels are alarmingly high and are therefore responsible for increasing the stress and anxiety felt by the patient. Various pharmacological and non-pharmacological approaches have been developed, but premedication remains the most widely used. However, because of its undesirable effects, various studies have tried to find an alternative, in particular TM. TM is a non-pharmacological, risk-free and low-cost approach, and has been shown to be effective in several studies.The aim of our study was to evaluate the contribution of TM on perioperative anxiety during scheduled orthopaedic surgery of the lower limb under AR. To achieve this objective, we conducted a prospective randomised controlled trial in the orthopaedic operating theatre, including 104 patients proposed for scheduled orthopaedic surgery of the lower limb under AR. Patients were randomised by computerised randomisation software into two groups:

- **Study group (M):** patients in this group listened to the music of their choice via headphones during the procedure.
- **Control group (T):** the patients in this group wore headphones without music and were therefore naturally exposed to the sounds of the operating theatre without any isolation.

The primary endpoint was to evaluate the effectiveness of music therapy in managing perioperative anxiety. The secondary endpoints were postoperative pain, intraoperative haemodynamic stability and patient satisfaction. Post-operatively, the mean VAS anxiety scores of group M were statistically significantly lower than those of group T. The mean VAS pain scores at H2 and H6 post-op in group M were statistically significantly lower than in group T. The time to first analgesic treatment was significantly longer in patients in group M than in group T. We noted a significant difference between the two groups at all times of intraoperative HR measurement, except at T10 when we did not note a significant difference in HR between the 2 groups. The mean values of PAS and PAD observed intraoperatively were comparable in the two groups, although the values of PAS and PAD were lower in group M at all times of measurement. The mean FRs observed intraoperatively were comparable in the two groups, except at T60 and T80 where we found a significant difference between the 2 groups. In addition, the mean FRs measured at all times were lower in the M group than in the T group.

Post-operatively, the satisfaction rate of group M was significantly higher than that of group T. When asked if they wanted to repeat the procedure using the same protocol, we found a highly significant difference in favour of group M. At the end of this study, TM proved to be an effective approach for combating perioperative anxiety. It led to a reduction in postoperative anxiety and pain scores, a significant reduction in intraoperative heart rate and an increase in patient satisfaction.Our results are therefore encouraging, and argue in favour of the value of MT for orthopaedic surgery of the lower limb under AR. Its cost Its low dosage and ease of use mean that it can be used in operating theatres as a non-pharmacological anxiolytic.

REFERENCES

1. Wilson CJ, Mitchelson AJ, Tzeng TH, El-Othmani MM, Saleh J, Vasdev S, et al. Caring for the surgically anxious patient: a review of the interventions and a guide to optimizing surgical outcomes. Am J Surg. Jul 2016;212(1):151-9.

2. Székely A, Balog P, Benkö E, Breuer T, Székely J, Kertai MD, et al. Anxiety Predicts Mortality and Morbidity After Coronary Artery and Valve Surgery-A 4-Year Follow-Up Study. Psychosom Med. Sept 2007;69(7):625-31.

3. Rymaszewska J, Kiejna A, Hadryś T. Depression and anxiety in coronary artery bypass grafting patients. Eur Psychiatry. June 2003;18(4):155-60.

4. Mackenzie JW. Daycase anaesthesia and anxiety A study of anxiety profiles amongst patients attending a Day Bed Unit. Anaesthesia. May 1989;44(5):437-40.

5. Kracht JM, Busch-Vishniac IJ, West JE. Noise in the operating rooms of Johns Hopkins Hospital. J Acoust Soc Am. 1 May 2007;121(5):2673-80.

6. Giannoudis PV, Dinopoulos H, Chalidis B, Hall GM. Surgical stress response. Injury. Dec 2006;37:S3-9.

7. Koelsch S, Fuermetz J, Sack U, Bauer K, Hohenadel M, Wiegel M, et al. Effects of Music Listening on Cortisol Levels and Propofol Consumption during Spinal Anesthesia. Front Psychol. 2011;11(5):263-82.

8. Beydon L, Rouxel A, Camut N, Schinkel N, Malinovsky JM, Aveline C, et al. Sedative premedication before surgery - A multicentre randomized study versus placebo. Anaesth Crit Care Pain Med. June 2015;34(3):165-71.

9. Maurice-Szamburski A, Auquier P, Viarre-Oreal V, Cuvillon P, Carles M, Ripart J, et al. Effect of Sedative Premedication on Patient Experience After General Anesthesia: A Randomized Clinical Trial. JAMA. March 3, 2015;313(9):916.

10. Jaruzel CB, Kelechi TJ. Relief from anxiety using complementary therapies in the perioperative period: A principle-based concept analysis. Complement Ther Clin Pract. August 2016;24:1-5.

11. Lecourt É. La musicothérapie. Paris: Éditions Eyrolles; 2019;36(977):190-1.

12. Conrad C. Music for healing: from magic to medicine. The Lancet. Dec 2010;376(9757):1980-1.

13. Lecourt É. Découvrir la musicothérapie. Paris: Eyrolles; 2005;40(977):190-1.

14. Caumo W, Schmidt AP, Schneider CN, Bergmann J, Iwamoto CW, Adamatti LC, et al. Risk factors for postoperative anxiety in adults: Postoperative anxiety in adults. Anaesthesia. August 2001;56(8):720-8.

15. Guidelines for community noise. World Health Organization. Occupational

and Environmental Health Team. (1999). Guidelines for community noise. World Health Organization. 1999;56(8):30-8.

16. Katz JD. Noise in the Operating Room. Anesthesiology. 1 Oct 2014;121(4):894-8.

17. Hodge B, Thompson JF. Noise pollution in the operating theatre. The Lancet. Apr 1990;335(8694):891-4.

18. Shapiro RA, Berland T. Noise in the Operating Room. N Engl J Med. 14 Dec 1972;287(24):1236-8.

19. Gómez Gallego M, Gómez García J. Musicoterapia en la enfermedad de Alzheimer: efectos cognitivos, psicológicos y conductuales. Neurología. June 2017;32(5):300-8.

20. Geretsegger M, Elefant C, Mössler KA, Gold C. Music therapy for people with autism spectrum disorder. Cochrane Developmental, Psychosocial and Learning Problems Group, editor. Cochrane Database Syst Rev . 17 June 2014;2016(3):100-5.

21. Sharda M, Tuerk C, Chowdhury R, Jamey K, Foster N, Custo-Blanch M, et al. Music improves social communication and auditory-motor connectivity in children with autism. Transl Psychiatry. 23 Oct 2018;8(1):231.

22. Li Y, Xing X, Shi X, Yan P, Chen Y, Li M, et al. The effectiveness of music therapy for patients with cancer: A systematic review and meta-analysis. J Adv Nurs. May 2020;76(5):1111-23.

23. Santiváñez-Acosta R, Tapia-López EDLN, Santero M. Music Therapy in Pain and Anxiety Management during Labor: A Systematic Review and Meta-Analysis. Medicina (Mex). 10 Oct 2020;56(10):526.

24. Gokyildiz Surucu S, Ozturk M, Avcibay Vurgec B, Alan S, Akbas M. The effect of music on pain and anxiety of women during labour on first time pregnancy: A study from Turkey. Complement Ther Clin Pract. Feb 2018;30:96-102.

25. Wu PY, Huang ML, Lee WP, Wang C, Shih WM. Effects of music listening on anxiety and physiological responses in patients undergoing awake craniotomy. Complement Ther Med. June 2017;32:56-60.

26. Kahloul M, Mhamdi S, Nakhli MS, Sfeyhi AN, Azzaza M, Chaouch A, et al. Effects of music therapy under general anesthesia in patients undergoing abdominal surgery. Libyan J Med. jan 2017;12(1):1260886.

27. Binns-Turner PG, Wilson LL, Pryor ER, Boyd GL, Prickett CA. Perioperative music and its effects on anxiety, hemodynamics, and pain in women undergoing mastectomy. AANA J. August 2011;79(4 Suppl):S21-27.

28. Bashiri M, Akcali D, Coskun D. Evaluation of pain and patient satisfaction by music therapy in patients with endoscopy/colonoscopy. Turk J Gastroenterol.

August 31, 2018;29(5):574-9.

29. Hauck M, Metzner S, Rohlffs F, Lorenz J, Engel AK. The influence of music and music therapy on pain- induced neuronal oscillations measured by magnetencephalography. Pain. Apr 2013;154(4):539-47.

30. Nilsson U. The Anxiety- and Pain-Reducing Effects of Music Interventions: A Systematic Review. AORN J. Apr 2008;87(4):780-807.

31. Johnston K, Rohaly-Davis J. An introduction to music therapy: Helping the oncology patient in the ICU: Crit Care Nurs Q. Feb 1996;18(4):54-60.

32. Bettermann H, Amponsah D, Cysarz D, Van Leeuwen P. Musical rhythms in heart period dynamics: a cross- cultural and interdisciplinary approach to cardiac rhythms. Am J Physiol-Heart Circ Physiol. 1 Nov 1999;277(5):H1762-70.

33. Kindler CH, Harms C, Amsler F, Ihde-Scholl T, Scheidegger D. The Visual Analog Scale Allows Effective Measurement of Preoperative Anxiety and Detection of Patients' Anesthetic Concerns: Anesth Analg. March 2000;90(3):706-12.

34. Azi LMT de A, Azi ML, Viana MM, Panont ALP, Oliveira RMF, Sadigursky D, et al. Benefits of intraoperative music on orthopedic surgeries under spinal anesthesia: A randomized clinical trial. Complement Ther Med. Dec 2021;63:102777.

35. Kaur H, Saini N, Singh G, Singh A, Dahuja A, Kaur R. Music as an aid to Allay Anxiety in Patients Undergoing Orthopedic Surgeries under Spinal Anesthesia. Noise Health. 2022;24(112):7-12.

36. Kukreja P, Talbott K, MacBeth L, Ghanem E, Sturdivant AB, Woods A, et al. Effects of Music Therapy During Total Knee Arthroplasty Under Spinal Anesthesia: A Prospective Randomized Controlled Study. Cureus . March 24, 2020;30(4):100-20.

37. Wang Y, Dong Y, Li Y. Perioperative Psychological and Music Interventions in Elderly Patients Undergoing Spinal Anesthesia: Effect on Anxiety, Heart Rate Variability, and Postoperative Pain. Yonsei Med J. 2014;55(4):1101.

38. Kühlmann AYR, De Rooij A, Kroese LF, Van Dijk M, Hunink MGM, Jeekel J. Meta-analysis evaluating music interventions for anxiety and pain in surgery. Br J Surg. 14 May 2018;105(7):773-83.

39. Cimen SG, Oğuz E, Gundogmus AG, Cimen S, Sandikci F, Ayli MD. Listening to music during arteriovenous fistula surgery alleviates anxiety: A randomized single-blind clinical trial. World J Transplant. 29 Apr 2020;10(4):79-89.

40. Zhang Z sheng, Wang X lin, Xu C liang, Zhang C, Cao Z, Xu W dong, et al. Music Reduces Panic: An Initial Study of Listening to Preferred Music

Improves Male Patient Discomfort and Anxiety During Flexible Cystoscopy. J Endourol. June 2014;28(6):739-44.

41. Jaber S, Bahloul H, Guétin S, Chanques G, Sebbane M, Eledjam JJ. Effects of non-sedation music therapy in intensive care patients undergoing ventilatory weaning versus non-ventilated patients. Ann Fr Anesth Réanimation. Jan 2007;26(1):30-8.

42. Ip HYV, Abrishami A, Peng PWH, Wong J, Chung F. Predictors of Postoperative Pain and Analgesic Consumption. Anesthesiology. 1 Sep 2009;111(3):657-77.

43. Angioli R, De Cicco Nardone C, Plotti F, Cafà EV, Dugo N, Damiani P, et al. Use of Music to Reduce Anxiety during Office Hysteroscopy: Prospective Randomized Trial. J Minim Invasive Gynecol. May 2014;21(3):454-9.

44. Gallagher LM, Gardner V, Bates D, Mason S, Nemecek J, DiFiore JB, et al. Impact of Music Therapy on Hospitalized Patients Post-Elective Orthopaedic Surgery: A Randomized Controlled Trial. Orthop Nurs. March 2018;37(2):124-33.

45. Steelman VM. Intraoperative Music Therapy. AORN J. Nov 1990;52(5):1026-34.

46. Kaur H, Shukla V, Bansal GL, Harsh HK, Joseph A, Bharadwaj MS. Extra note of music in anaesthesia. Int J Res Med Sci. 25 Jul 2019;7(8):3219.

47. Kalyani Np, Poonam Gg, Shalini Kt. Impact of intraoperative music therapy on the anaesthetic requirement and stress response in laparoscopic surgeries under general anaesthesia. Ain-Shams J Anaesthesiol. 2015;8(4):580.

48. Ilkkaya NK, Ustun FE, Sener EB, Kaya C, Ustun YB, Koksal E, et al. The Effects of Music, White Noise, and Ambient Noise on Sedation and Anxiety in Patients Under Spinal Anesthesia During Surgery. J Perianesth Nurs. oct 2014;29(5):418-26.

49. Gökçek E, Kaydu A. The effects of music therapy in patients undergoing septorhinoplasty surgery under general anaesthesia. Braz J Otorhinolaryngol. July 2020;86(4):419-26.

APPENDICES

APPENDIX 1

American Society of Anesthesiologists (ASA) classification Class I: patient in good health.

Class II: patients with moderate impairment of a major function.

Class III: patient with severe impairment o f a major function which does not result in disability.

Class IV: patient with severe impairment of a major function presenting a permanent threat to life.

Class V: moribund patient.

Class VI: brain-dead patient.

Visual Analogue Scale VAS: Anxiety

The EVA comes in the form of a 10 cm plastic ruler graduated in mm, which can be presented to the patient horizontally or vertically. On the face presented to the patient, there is a cursor that he or she moves along a straight line, one end of which corresponds to "No anxiety" and the other to "Maximum anxiety imaginable".Along this line, the patient must position the cursor at the point that best represents his or her anxiety. On the other side, there are millimetre scales seen only by the carer. The position of the cursor moved by the patient is used to read the intensity of anxiety, which is measured in mm.

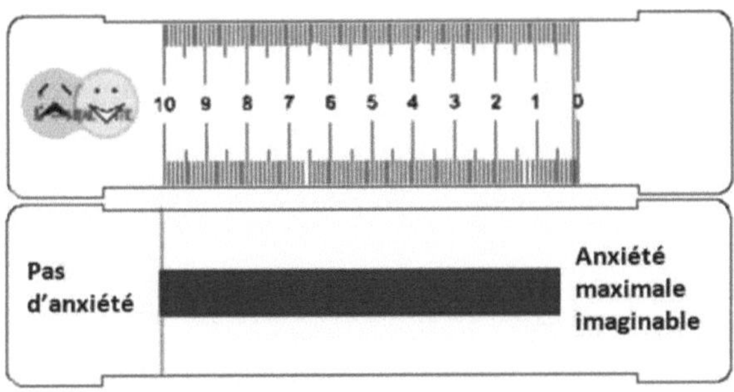

APPENDIX 3

Visual Analogue Scale VAS: Pain

The EVA comes in the form of a 10 cm plastic ruler graduated in mm, which can be presented to the patient horizontally or vertically.On the face presented to the patient, there is a cursor that he or she moves along a straight line, one end of which corresponds to "No pain" and the other to "Maximum imaginable pain".Along this line, the patient should position the cursor at the point that best locates the pain. On the other side, there are millimetre scales that can only be seen by the carer. The position of the cursor moved by the patient is used to read the intensity of the pain, which is measured in mm.

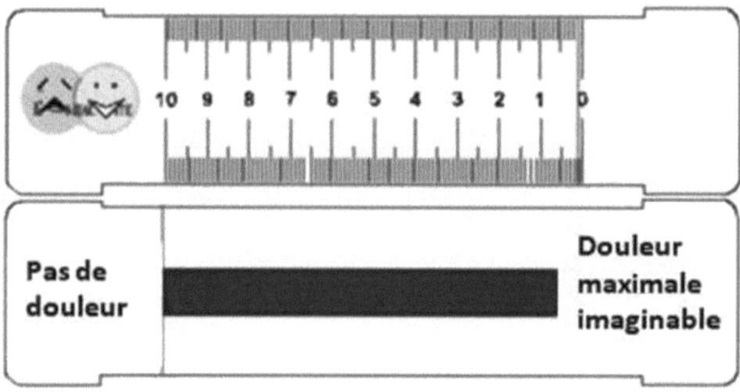

APPENDIX 4

موافقة المريض على اجراء بحث علمي

أهمية العلاج بالموسيقى في إدارة المرضى المقترحين لجراحة العظام في الطرف السفلي تحت التخدير الشوكي

إلى المريض انقه (إم وقف المشارك)

أقبل بالمشاركة في مشروع البحث بعنوان:

سيفي في إدارة المرضى المقترحين لدراحة العظام في الطرف السفلي تحت التخدير الشوكي

الوآتي :

- اطلعت على رسالة إلعلام المتعلقة بمشروع البحث المذكور رأعلاه

- تحصلت على معلومات واضحة مع الأجوبة على أسئلتي بخصوص مشروع البحث

- لقد ث كرهعالمي شفاهيًا ركتابيً بأهداف المشروع وطرق جمع البيانات وأشكال مشاركتي في المشروع من قبل الباحث .

كماد كرهعالمي أيضا بـ :

- فريقا تأمين التغاطي لمزايا المعطيات التي تخصني

- على بصائي مشاركت ملطر عاد في الانسحاب في أي وقت ثراد منلهب كًا دون أن يتسبب لي ذلك في أي ضرر .

- ح ق بي ، لو النصال الخطار بالباحث الرابسي عندما تكون لي أسئلة حول مشروع البحث

وعلى ذلك :

كامنحت أجال كافيا للتخاذ قرار في خصوص المشاركة في مشروع البحث أقبل بكل حرية رسمية قرمياً أن تكون معطياتي الشخصية الخاصة بالبحث أر معطيات الشخص تحت وأبقي متلحة إلى المسؤولين على البحث وعند الضرورة إلى السلطات الصحية على ثم معالجة تلك المعطيات في كنف احترام السر الطبي مع إخفاء هويّتي .

الإمضاء

Bromage score

Modified Bromage score
1 complete engine block
2 engine block almost complete (moves feet)
3 partial block (moves feet and knees)
4 detectable weakness in hip flexion
5 no hip weakness when lying down
6 Knee bend standing with support

7 Knee bend, standing without support Sheet N :

APPENDIX 6

Personnel number :

Full name :

Date :

Pre-operational data :

Age	Gender	Weight	Size	BMI
Level of education: illiterate/ primary/ secondary/ university				
Marital status: married/ divorced/ single/ widowed				
History:				
ASA :				
EVA anxiety :				

Intraoperative data :

	T0 (before RA)	T10	T20	T30	T40	T50	T60	T70	T80	T90	T100	T110	T120
FC													
NOT													
PAD													
FR													

Type of surgery :	Sensitive block installation time :	Duration of anaesthesia :
Duration of surgery :	Engine block installation time :	Dose of ephedrine administered:

Postoperative data :

EVA anxiety :	
EVA pain at H2 post-op :	EVA pain at H6 post-op :
Time to first analgesic :	
Satisfaction (1: very satisfied; 2: satisfied; 3: undetermined; 4: not satisfied)	
Would you like to repeat the procedure using the same protocol? : yes: no	

SUMMARY

PROBLEM :

Surgery and anaesthesia are two experiences that are generally poorly received by patients, increasing stress and anxiety and potentially hampering the quality of perioperative care. This anxiety is heightened in orthopaedic surgery, where noise levels are alarmingly high. Several alternatives are used to manage this anxiety. Music therapy, a non-pharmacological approach, has been shown to be effective in reducing perioperative stress.

PURPOSE OF THE WORK :

To evaluate the contribution of music therapy during orthopaedic surgery of the lower limb under spinal anaesthesia on the management of patient anxiety.

PATIENTS AND METHODS :

After obtaining informed consent from the patients, we conducted a single-centre, prospective, randomised, single-blind clinical trial in the Anaesthesia and Intensive Care Department in collaboration with the Orthopaedics Department of the Habib BOURGUIBA University Hospital in Sfax. We included patients classified ASA I and II proposed for scheduled surgery of the lower limb under AR. They were divided into two equivalent groups: group M who listened to music through headphones during surgery and group T who wore headphones without music. The primary endpoint was the management of perioperative anxiety. The secondary endpoints were intraoperative haemodynamic variations, postoperative pain and patient satisfaction.

RESULTS:

One hundred and four patients were included and randomised into two groups of 52. Demographic parameters, comorbidities, duration of surgery and time to onset of sensory and motor block were comparable between the two groups. Postoperative VAS anxiety values were significantly lower in group M than in group T. Postoperative pain VAS values at H2 and H6 were significantly lower in group M than in group T. The time to first analgesic request was longer in group M than in group T. We noted a significant difference between the two groups at all times of intraoperative HR measurement except at T10 where we did not note a significant difference in

HR between the 2 groups. However, we did not show a statistically significant difference in PAS, PAD and RF between the 2 groups. Patient satisfaction was better in group M with a statistically significant difference compared to group T.

CONCLUSION:

Music therapy is proving to be an effective approach to managing perioperative anxiety. It has been shown to reduce anxiety levels, reduce perceived postoperative pain, stabilise intraoperative heart rate and improve patient satisfaction.

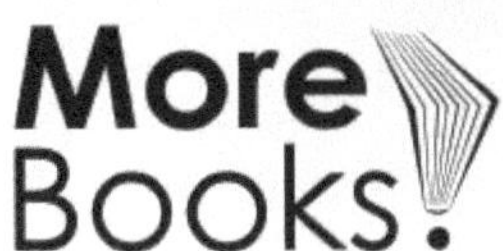

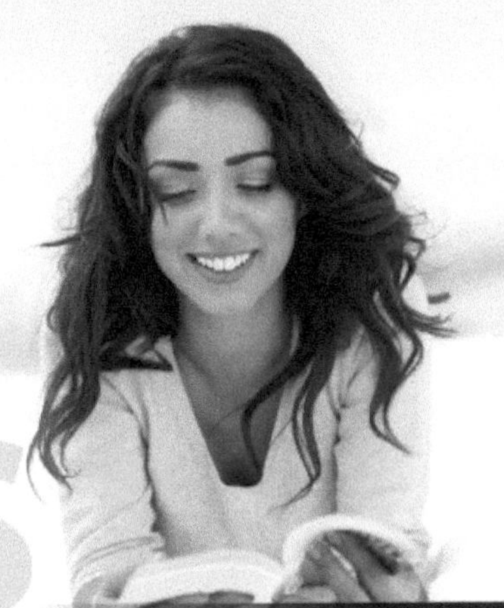

I want morebooks!

Buy your books fast and straightforward online - at one of world's fastest growing online book stores! Environmentally sound due to Print-on-Demand technologies.

Buy your books online at
www.morebooks.shop

Kaufen Sie Ihre Bücher schnell und unkompliziert online – auf einer der am schnellsten wachsenden Buchhandelsplattformen weltweit! Dank Print-On-Demand umwelt- und ressourcenschonend produziert.

Bücher schneller online kaufen
www.morebooks.shop

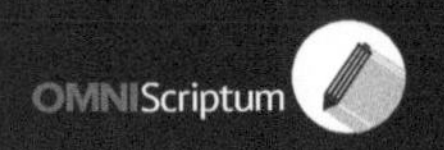

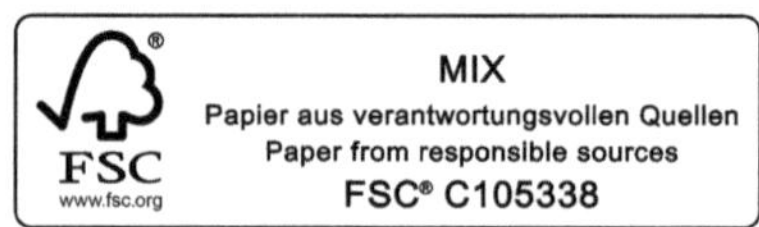

Printed by Books on Demand GmbH, Norderstedt / Germany